# Six Lies

# Women Believe

# About Their Health

LESA M. LAWSON, ND

# DEDICATION

**T**o my mom, Herma Lawson, and grandmother, Mabel Smith, whose knowledge of herbs made them steep remedies for whatever ailed my childhood afflictions. The knowledge that they instilled in me is unsurpassed by anything else that I have learnt because their teaching was and is, infused with love.

I am so grateful to my sisters, Charmaine and Althea for their encouragement and studied urging in the completion of this work. Motivation is a wonderful thing.

## Let It Be Understood

The standard disclaimer is simply this: the information contained in this book is not intended to provide medical advice nor should it take the place of medical treatment from your own physician.

That disclaimer, however, is antithetical to my purpose. I have written to encourage people to think critically and do for themselves what no physician can do.

The author does not take responsibility for any consequence from any remedy or application of supplements, herbs or preparations by any person reading the information in this book.

For every woman who is on the cusp of discovery: may your journey be filled with wonder.

May you embrace true selflessness in the midst of strength, and find your freedom.

# Table of Contents

## MEET SUPERWOMAN

If you were to review the average mother's unofficial resume, you might think that she's an octopus because of the job titles that she holds:

- ✓ Chemist
- ✓ Plumber
- ✓ Seamstress
- ✓ Cook
- ✓ Designer

- ✓ Teacher
- ✓ Doctor
- ✓ Carpenter
- ✓ Retrieval Service
- ✓ Policewoman

to name just a few.

Just because she doesn't tote these titles on a sheet of vellum does not mean that they aren't very much parts of who she is.

Mom works to provide for herself and her family; she drives or takes the train or bus, and is sometimes jostled or harangued all day. She arrives home, after having stopped for groceries or medicine, and begins her third job of the day, the first having been the morning routine.

Now, she has children with whom she must commiserate. She needs to listen, encourage and correct, prepare a meal, check homework, prepare or supervise baths for young ones; and there are bedtime routines, where, if she's not careful, she may doze during the prayers. Setting the kitchen to rights is next on the agenda, and then come all the other little things that need to be done. In many instances, the only self-care that she performed was to change her clothes and wash her hands before preparing dinner. By the way, hubby is still waiting his turn.

This lifestyle is the norm, give or take a scenario, for many working moms, single or married. Thank God for husbands who help and share the responsibilities of the home; we truly honor them, and do not take them for granted. In our changing society, however, this happens on a lesser scale. Many women work themselves to the bone, alone.

While mom is caring and cleaning and cooking, she orders priorities in her life. Sitting atop the mountain are her children and husband, if there is one. She tends to their comfort because she loves them. Their illness, health, sadness, joys, failures and successes are all hers.

In the middle of this, is her job because she needs it. Overtime, if required, must be done; a good performance review is contingent upon her dedication and focus. Her friends and external family are next in line. Needs are there, too.

Her faith is next, if she is spiritually-minded, and she may have church obligations. Last and certainly least, is herself; she brings up the rear. Her health, happiness, stress levels, feelings… yes, her life comes last.

Is it not rather ironic that she places her needs last, considering that she is such a strong force upon which so many people and things rely? I am, in no way, placing the role of woman above that of man. Unfortunately, our society has become so harsh, that more and more women have had to add additional roles to that which we were originally given. Some cannot be helped, and some are self-appointed.

Sadly, the more that we add to our lives, the less that we subtract from them. The result is that we are more overworked, tired, stressed, irritable, and ill than we need to be.

A woman's self-care is dependent upon the precepts that she has come to accept. As she mentally rehearses them, she repeats them until, soon, the precepts become personal beliefs that she begins to teach other women, including her own daughters.

She perpetuates the lie. We all do.

All this has made us fearful, unhappy, booby-trapped women who are imprisoned in a cage without bars. I decided that I will no longer live in this way. Will you join me?

Let us expose the lies that we have been taught to believe, and free ourselves from these bondages, forever.

*What meds are these that shape our dreams;*
*that keep us bound; elicit screams*
*with side-effects of varied themes*
*and more meds so debilitating?*

## LIE NUMBER 1

### IT IS NATURAL TO REQUIRE MEDICATION, AS WE GROW OLDER.

In many instances, when we visit the doctor in our late thirties and later years, we begin to hear certain statements that form parentheses around our blood-work or routine test results. On occasion, a client or relative will tell me that the test results showed elevated blood pressure or cholesterol, but her doctor said that "it's normal for her age." Well, how does that make sense? What is it about her age that triggered an elevation in blood pressure?

The doctor may also say that that blood pressure becomes elevated with age and that medication will take care of it.

Unfortunately, doctors sometimes neglect to tell their patients that blood pressure medication is a life-long drug habit. Once started on it, one needs to stay on it. Why? The medication does not fix the problem; it is a pacifier. Blood pressure medications tend to thin the blood, so that it will pass through a smaller, still-clogged blood vessel or artery. Can you see the problem that remains? You're right – the blood vessel or artery is still clogged. The problem remains.

If the problem has not been fixed, then it makes sense that it will worsen, over time and the thing that we fear may happen. One side-effect of blood pressure medications on a long-term basis is heart attack. Why? Some meds have or are calcium channel blockers; that is, they relax blood vessels by stopping calcium from entering cells. The body needs calcium. Your heart needs calcium. Fix the real problem, instead of blocking something that the heart actually needs.

In addition, blood pressure meds usually come in twos or threes. Taking more than one medicine may change the way in which your body absorbs or uses a drug. Chances are that the diet has not really changed, so different foods or alcohol may also change the way in which a drug acts in your body.

Here are some other common side effects of blood pressure medications, according to the National Institutes of Health[1]

Some common side effects of high blood pressure medicines include:

- Cough
- Diarrhea or constipation
- Dizziness or lightheadedness
- Erection problems
- Feeling nervous
- Feeling tired, weak, drowsy, or a lack of energy
- Headache
- Nausea or vomiting
- Skin rash
- Weight loss or gain without trying

Another issue is that many of these medicines are diuretics; that means that they pull

---

[1] High blood pressure medicines, U.S. Department of Health and Human Services, https://medlineplus.gov/ency/article/007484.htm

water from the body and increase urination. Greater urination can lead to dehydration, especially if the patient is not replenishing her water intake. Dehydration then leads to joint pain, headaches and constipation, among other things.

Many physicians believe that high blood pressure cannot be overcome. Because of this belief, they prescribe blood pressure medications as a stop gap. For some patients the medication does help to keep some symptoms at bay; however, this demonstrates the proverbial 'finger in the dyke' mentality. The side effects multiply one condition into three or four different ones.

This philosophy of needing medication to make our aging easier is missing a vital component. What is it that causes people to need drugs in the first place? Is it not usually because of poor diet (including hydration), rest, exercise habits, and too much stress? Who decided to justify our poor self-treatment with the old age excuse? If you are a believer in God and the Bible and you believe the 'older = meds' philosophy, show me the proof in the Bible. If you are not a believer, you are not off the hook; show me your proof.

It would make sense to take a few steps back to the root of the problem. Now, please note that I am not stating that people ought not to take medications. Sometimes, a condition is dire or has so worsened because of lack of care, that regulatory emergency measures need to be taken. The patient may need to be kept from dying by medicated measures. Once the beep on the machine becomes a little less erratic, however, that lady needs to go into battle mode and fight for her life.

Fighting means that while returning to the root, we examine the causes that brought us to this stage in the first place, and reverse them. This is called taking ownership, followed by stewardship.

Reversal includes dietary changes, proper hydration with pure water, exercise (gradual, at first), and rest. Periodic short cleanses and a longer detox program won't hurt, either. A twice-yearly whole-body detoxification rids the body of harmful toxins, alleviates cravings and can even jump-start the unclogging of arteries and veins.

If you do not know what to do about detoxification or how to do it properly, seek help. If you have never done one and you are ill, you want to ensure that you do not further harm yourself when toxins begin to be released from the cells of your body. You will need to eliminate some things but at the end of your process, you will feel

yourself getting better.

*Pain in the fingers and pain in the heart*
*HDL, LDL, where should you start?*
*High sugar levels make fingertips sting*
*Let these top the list of your least favorite things*

## LIE NUMBER 2

### HIGH BLOOD PRESSURE, HIGH CHOLESTEROL, DIABETES, AND ARTHRITIS ARE NORMAL, WITH AGE.

This is a notion that some doctors actually entertain, and, unfortunately, they pass this depressing, paralyzing information on to their patients. Soon, if we're not careful, too many of us will be 'drinking the Kool-Aid'. How can this even be considered normal? Let us look at this lie closely.

## Definitions

**High blood pressure:** a common disorder in which blood pressure remains abnormally high (a reading of 140/90 mm Hg or greater).

*www.wordnetweb.princeton.edu/perl/webwn*

**High cholesterol:** A familial disorder that is characterized by an extremely high concentration of cholesterol in the blood and cells. *www.thefreedictionary.com*

**Diabetes:** A disorder of the metabolism, causing excessive thirst and the production of large amounts of urine. The metabolism is a collection of chemical reactions that takes place in the body's cells. Metabolism converts the fuel in the food we eat into the energy needed to power everything we do, from moving to thinking to growing. *www.memidex.com/diabetes+polygenic- disorder*

**Arthritis**: Arthritis (from Greek arthro-, joint + -itis, inflammation; plural: arthritides) is a form of joint disorder that involves inflammation of one or more joints. *Central Florida Health and Wellness Magazine. http://healthandwellnessfl.com/arthritis-and-joint-pain/*

What is the common word in these definitions? **Disorder**

The word, disorder, according to the Merriam Webster dictionary means "to disturb the order of;" or "to disturb the regular or normal functions of."

If something has a particular order or normal pattern and that order has been disturbed, it stands to reason that the original pattern is lying in a forgotten heap, somewhere. We need to return to it and it does not need to be an expensive journey. In fact, returning to the original pattern is cheaper than surgery, hospitalizations, or a life-time's supply of medications.

The accepted norms for blood pressure are:

- <u>Normal</u>: Less than 120/80

- <u>Pre-hypertension</u>: 120-139/80-89

- <u>Stage 1 high blood pressure</u>: 140-159/90-99

- <u>Stage 2 high blood pressure</u>: 160 and above/100 and above

There are plants, herbs, and essential oils that can be used in the process of normalizing blood pressure. One solution is drinking garlic tea: crush two garlic cloves, remove trash, and add garlic to a pot with 10 ounces of pure water. Simmer for about 10 to 15 minutes. You can add a little raw honey, but it is good to drink as is.

Another method is to add 6-10 cloves of garlic (skin removed) to a bottle of Bragg's apple cider vinegar. Re-cap the bottle and let it sit for at least four days. Take 1-2 tablespoons in 8-10 ounces of water, daily, for 4-6 weeks. Take either early in the morning or last thing at night.

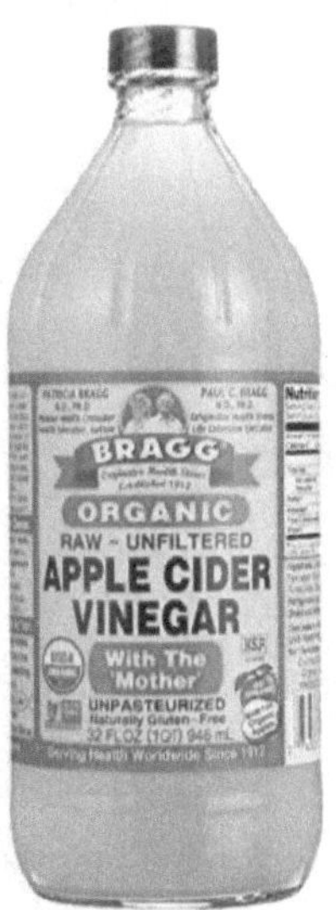

Breadfruit leaf tea is another great remedy.

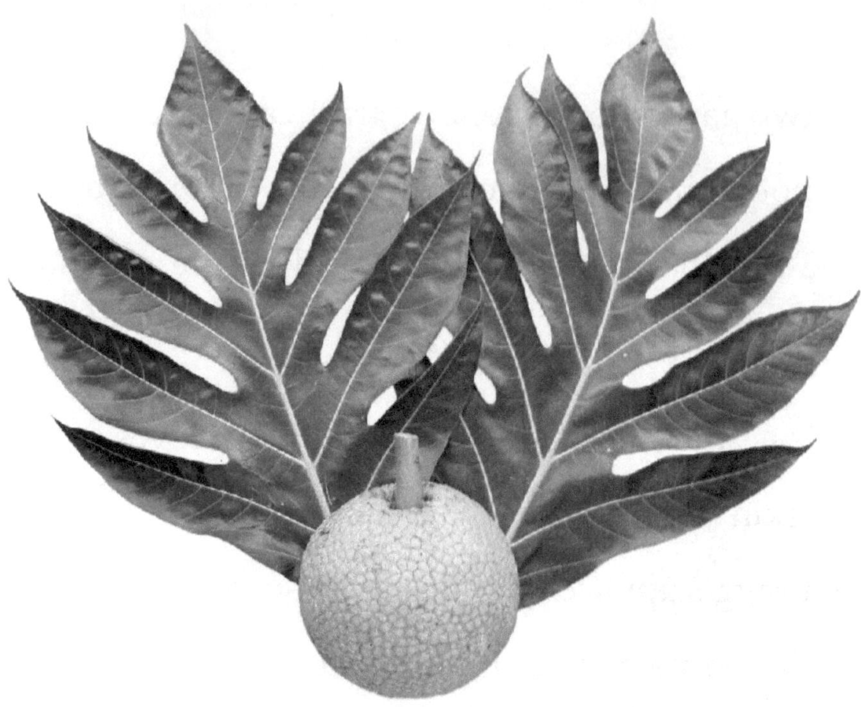

If you are familiar with the breadfruit, you can have an even more potent tea if you add one

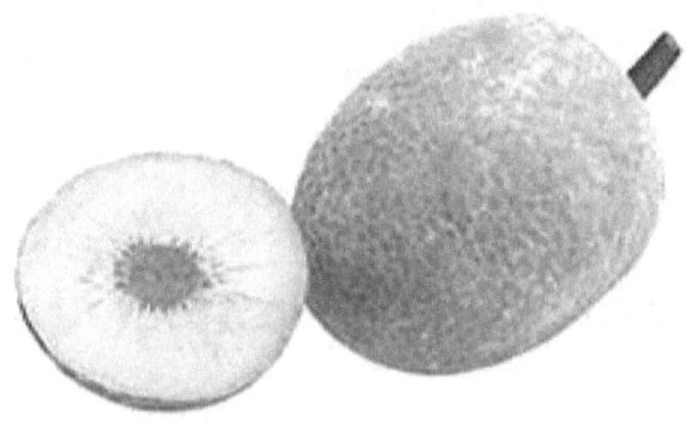

chopped, breadfruit leaf (dried or fresh) to the simmering garlic water, and drink while hot. For dried leaves, boil for 15 minutes; if green, steep the leaves in the hot garlic water (first simmer the garlic, then add the breadfruit leaf after removing the pot from the fire.) Cover and let sit for 10 minutes). [2]

Blending cucumber and garlic is also an excellent remedy.

There are other natural herbs, oils, and spices that help to lower blood pressure. Cayenne pepper is one such warrior. It is a wonderful spice that I use quite frequently. According to the editors of Consumer Guide, cayenne pepper is a "popular home treatment for mild high blood pressure. [It]

---

[2] Breadfruit tree preparation is believed to lower hypertension and treat taeniasis (a digestive tract infection caused by tapeworms), diabetes, sore eyes, sciatica, enlarged spleen, skin infections, boils, burns, gout, and rheumatism. Leaf extracts have been used to treat toothaches and diarrhea. *http://www.naturalstandard.com*

allows smooth blood flow by preventing platelets from clumping together and accumulating in the blood." [3] Sprinkle cayenne over cooked foods or add it during cooking. You can also add one-eighth teaspoon of cayenne pepper to a jar with eight ounces of water and the juice of one-half fresh lemon. Drink on an empty stomach.

Bananas, because of their high levels of potassium, are also blood pressure reducers. The potassium in bananas, ripe or green, can counter salt intake. Of course, this does not release anyone to eat a lot of salt and then eat bananas. The average person requires about three to four servings of

---

[3] Editors of Consumer Guide. "Home Remedies for High Blood Pressure" 22 January 2007. HowStuffWorks.com. http://health.howstuffworks.com/wellness/natural-medicine/home-remedies/home-remedies-for-high-blood-pressure.htm. 19 June 2013

potassium-rich foods, daily. The 2010 Dietary Guidelines for Americans suggest that people with hypertension should increase their potassium intake to about 4,700 milligrams.[4]

The BBC news reported on a study that was performed by Kasturba Medical College in Manipal, Southern India. The study, which involved human volunteers, showed that two bananas a day can help control high blood pressure, offering a cheap alternative to expensive drugs, according to scientists.[5] A banana has 422 milligrams. Note that green bananas need to be boiled, baked or roasted.

Other potassium food sources include boiled

---

[4] http://www.health.gov/dietaryguidelines/dga2010/ dietaryguidelines2010.pdf

[5] http://news.bbc.co.uk/2/hi/health/264552.stm

or baked potatoes with the skin (hold the sour cream), non-sulfured dried apricots, currants, and raisins, orange juice (fresh squeezed), spinach, baked sweet potatoes, cantaloupe, and winter squash.

Let's look at some herbs and essential oils that support the heart and some corresponding organs and situations.

## Herbs that Support the Heart

Did you know that anemia can cause the heart to race? Some women may also experience shortness of breath, fainting, and chest pains, if anemia is very low. In cases of severe anemia, the blood oxygen levels can become so low that a person can have a heart attack.

The following herbs and herbal combinations are helpful and available from Nature's Sunshine[6].

**Anemia**: Chlorophyll, B-12 Complete, I-X

**Arthritis:** Calcium plus Vitamin D, Yucca, Relief Formula, EverFlex

**<u>Blood Pressure (high):</u>** Blood Pressurex, Kidney Activator, Nutri-Calm, Capsicum/Garlic/Parley

**Blood Pressure (low):** Master Gland formula, Herbal Trace Mineral

**Cholesterol:** Cholester-Reg II, Red Yeast Rice, Flax Seed Oil, Fat Grabber

**Diabetes:** Sugar-Reg, Blood Sugar Formula, Pro-Pancreas, Golden Seal

---

[6] www.naturessunshine.com

**Heart Health:** Cardio Assurance, Hawthorn Berries

**Essential Oils**

Pure essential oils are extracted from the leaves, fruit and bark of plants and are quite helpful to the body. Oils that are of therapeutic grade assure safe internal use. The essential oils produced by **Nature's Sunshine** and dōTERRA®* are of therapeutic grade and can also be applied topically, as well as used in a diffuser. Some people even use oils in cooking. If at all possible, use natural methods to support your body's healing and maintenance. Essential oils constitute one such method. Remember that each person is different and may respond differently to oils, and also at different speeds.

**Note:** Some essential oils are gentle and do not require dilution before topical application. Oils such as Lavender and Serenity fall within this category. Some oils are hotter (e.g. Cinnamon bark or Oregano), and should be diluted with coconut oil prior to being applied to the skin.

Always dilute oils when applying to children, unless you are rubbing the oils on the bottom of their feet. Consider the same strategy with sensitive individuals and the elderly.

***Order information for Nature's Sunshine and dōTERRA® essential oils is on the last page of this book.**

# Essential Oils and Blends for High Blood Pressure

## Oils:

Cassia

Frankincense

Helichrysum

Lavender

Lemon

Marjoram

Ylang Ylang

Clove

Eucalyptus

## Oil Blends:

Grounding Blend

Invigorating Blend

Clary Sage

Calming Blend

Wintergreen

## Protocol Suggestions[7]:

- Combine 3 drops each of Basil, Lavender, and Marjoram in a capsule, daily.

- Combine the following oils with 25 drops of coconut oil:

  4 drops Cassia

  4 drops Frankincense

  6 drops Helichrysum

  4 drops Marjoram

  6 drops Ylang Ylang

## Oil Application Suggestions:

Massage the blend onto the bottoms of the feet, on the wrists, the breast bone, over the heart, the carotid arteries, and the back of the neck.

---

[7] *Modern Essentials* and *Essentials of the Earth, 1st Edition.*

Add drops of oil to a diffuser and/or to your bath water (agitate the water often).

## Herbal Remedies to Lower High Cholesterol

We know that high cholesterol is directly related to one's diet and lifestyle. Keep a food diary and examine the things that you are putting into your mouth, including liquids, gum, and candy. Note your daily exercise, as well. You might be able to see the cause of your rising cholesterol before your doctor does.

There are herbs, essential oils, spices, and plants that are helpful in lowering cholesterol. Some include alfalfa leaf tea, almonds, bitter melon, carob, dandelion root tea, flax seeds (ground), Fo-ti, ginger, green tea, Hawthorn berry tea, oats, oat straw, pine nuts, pistachios, psyllium husk, pumpkin, sesame, and sunflower seeds. Do some research on the one that you would like to try or call me to sign up for your breakthrough program.

**Essential Oils and Blends for High Cholesterol:**

Cassia, Cypress, Lavender, Lemongrass, Rosemary, Basil, Helichrysum

**Essential oils based products:**

**dōTERRA**® Life Long Vitality Supplements (LLV). These include Omega 3s which are so vital to the heart.

**Suggested protocols:**

• Take an empty capsule and add 5-6 drops of Lemongrass, or Lemongrass with Cypress and Lavender, or Lemongrass with Cassia.

## Helpful Herbs for Diabetes

Bilberry, Bitter Melon, Chamomile, Cinnamon, Fenugreek, Ginseng, Holy Basil, and Prickly Pear Cactus (aka. tuna).

**Suggested protocol:** One teaspoon of bitter melon in a glass of water with the juice of ½ fresh lemon.

## Essential Oils for Diabetes

**Oils and Blends:** Grounding Blend, Basil, Coriander, Lavender, Protective Blend

**Essential Oils Based Products:**

dōTERRA® Vitality Supplements (LLV), TerraZyme

**Other Oils:** Cassia, Cinnamon, Clove, Cypress, Eucalyptus, Frankincense, Geranium, Helichrysum, Marjoram, Peppermint

**Suggested Protocols:**

Beneficial nutrition, rest, exercise, and the dōTERRA® Life Long Vitality Supplements (LLV) are quite helpful for all types of diabetes.

## Type 2

- Rub Grounding Blend on the feet in the morning

- Take 8-10 drops of Coriander and/or Basil in a capsule during the day. You may add 2 drops of Protective Blend to the capsule, as well.

- Rub Lavender on the feet, nightly.

If you are pre-diabetic, consider the following:

LLV supplements, GI Cleansing Formula/Probiotic Defense Formula cleanse and ongoing Detoxifying Blend.


## Herbs for Arthritis

**Burdock Root**  Make a tea, cook with it, or dry the root, grind and take in empty capsule.

**Flax**     Make a tea, strain and drink. Grind seeds and use in cereals and smoothies (If you suffer from a digestive condition, such as Irritable Bowel Syndrome (IBS), use flax oil instead of the seeds; the seeds may prove irritating to the system.)

**Turmeric**   Sprinkle on food, make a drink with fresh ginger, or take in capsules. Careful: turmeric stains!

**Nettles and Stinging Nettles**    Make a tea.

**Licorice** (do not use if you have high blood pressure, heart or kidney disease, or low potassium (hypokalemia).

## Essential Oils for Arthritis

**Oils and Blends:** Birch, Frankincense, Lavender, Lemon, Marjoram, Myrrh, Oregano, Peppermint, Soothing Blend, Vetiver, Wintergreen

**Essential oils based products:**

Soothing Blend Rub, GI Cleansing Formula, LifeLong Vitality Supplements (LLV)

**Other helpful Oils:** Eucalyptus, Geranium, German Chamomile, Ginger, Lime, and Sandalwood.

## Rheumatoid Arthritis:

**Temporary pain relief** – Apply Birch, Soothing Blend, Peppermint, Wintergreen, topically to affected areas. Use a carrier like fractionated coconut oil for those with sensitive skin. After application of oils, topically, use a heating pad for deeper penetration. Wintergreen should be diluted with carrier oil before topical application.

• Dr. David Hill, the Chief Medical Advisor to dōTERRA® referred to lemon and myrrh in his book, *Nature's Living Energy:*

"In treating patients with rheumatoid arthritis, I have found that a combination of Lemon and Myrrh, or Oregano applied topically can be quite soothing to inflamed joints."

He also recommends oils such as Cedarwood, Frankincense, Ginger, Myrrh and Ylang Ylang, in his book, *Frankincense*. He stated that these oils are heavy in sesquiterpenes which inhibit inflammatory response and, therefore, are helpful with arthritis.

• Add one drop of the Soothing Blend to the Soothing Blend Rub. Massage gently into painful areas.

• Equal drops of Wintergreen, Lemongrass, Frankincense, and Eucalyptus blended with a 50% carrier of coconut oil are recommended to be effective for arthritic pain.

For additional relief, use a local bath for the hands or feet. Fill a basin with hot water. Add 3-4 drops of the oil or blend and soak hands or feet, agitating the water often to keep the oils mixed with the water. Soak until the water begins to cool.

You may need to rotate between oils, over a period of time, in order to gain the most benefit. Some persons may take a longer time to experience a change, as we are all different. Of course, changing your diet, hydrating sufficiently, exercise and rest will all help with long term relief.

**Long term relief** – Some people have reported positive results by improving diet with the LifeLong Vitality supplements and/or using a cleansing protocol such as the GI Cleansing Formula cleansing protocol.

Many people live to ripe, old ages without being assaulted by the afore-mentioned afflictions. They actually take care of themselves by exercising, eating properly, hydrating, breathing deeply, getting good rest, cultivating a positive mindset, and living their lives purposefully. If you were to research the testimonies of the oldest living people around the world, you will find that they employed many of the life attitudes listed above.

I will give a little consideration to those doctors who believe that these ailments are normal with age. If a woman eats poorly, spends most of her existence sitting on her assurance instead of exercising, drinks more sugary drinks and alcohol than water, and just lives an unhealthy existence, then she will find herself expanding her family with relatives such as diabetes and high blood pressure. The term, hereditary or genetic diseases, in many instances, originates here, too. If your parent had heart disease and ate a poor diet, did not exercise, and adopted an unhealthy existence; and you have a similar diet and existence, the chances are that you will develop similar conditions.

Good health isn't hard; it just needs to become a habit. Think of it as you would your dream job. You have finally been hired and the pay rate is phenomenal. For the first three weeks, you're on your best behavior; you try to learn the ropes properly to impress your new boss and prevent you from stepping on anyone's toes. Usually, in a few weeks, if you're diligent, you learn the routine and become comfortable. *Habit*

*Today, Atkins diet, so I'll eat only meat*
*Next month, cabbage soup; size 6 is a feat*
*First, skinny, then fat, then skinny again*
*Oh, please, someone: get me off this gravy train!*

## Lie Number 3

### DIETING IS NORMAL AND IS THE ONLY EFFECTIVE WAY TO LOSE WEIGHT.

Poppycock! If dieting were the only way to lose weight and is normal, why do we not stick with it every day of our lives? Why do the effects of our diets not remain with many of us? Why do we have to keep dieting repeatedly?

Dieting ought not to be a way of life. It is like a stuck record, with you constantly returning to the scene of the crime, and there is no closure. I chuckled the first time I really paid attention to the first three letters of the word, **die**t. In truth, dieting has almost become a disorder, in itself. My definition of diet would be this:

*A common disorder, in which repetitive starvation robs the body of certain nutrients, produces temporary results and repeated deprivation.*

Emphasis on the word, disorder.

America's populace has reached its highest weight in history with one-half of us being overweight, and one-third, obese. Our culture's hype also affects our children; the media (and many of us) push them to develop distorted body images. May of our children are shamed and even forced into dieting at the tender age of nine or ten. Of course, we set them up for a life-time of disaster, with poor self-image, eating disorders, low self-esteem, and subconscious approval-seeking heading the list.

Our culture touts the latest diets to coerce us into achieving our desired weight, and people do *see* results (pun intended) – for a time. Unfortunately, these quick-fixes eventually backfire.

Truthfully, if you examine the health benefits, the level of permanence, and the degree of satisfaction, you would realize that diets don't work. Think about it; diets don't work because...

1) each person is unique, and each of us has different needs based on gender, age, ancestry and lifestyle. One diet, then, would not be right for everyone.

*2)* they are extreme solutions. Diets might work for a while, but research shows that almost all diets result in a 10-pound re-gain once they have ended. It makes sense that this would be the result. It's like holding your breath; eventually, your body will force you to seek air.

3) they are restrictive. Dieters who fail are not weak; our bodies need nourishment (and no, I don't mean Twinkies!). In many instances, the diet for quick results (and most of them are that) require nutrient restriction or the elimination of food groups. Now, if you are cleansing your body, that's another matter, entirely because you know that it is for a limited time, you're giving your body a respite, and dropping pounds is not your goal. Diets, by nature, require discipline and restriction at levels that a healthy human body cannot maintain for long periods of time.

4) most people see dieting as the only culprit and are disconnected from their reasons for gaining weight. Ignoring or discounting emotions, for instance, is often the first cause of weight imbalances.

Let us pick at this sore point for a bit. There's no one else here but you, me, and God. Take a notebook or write on the lines provided. Ask yourself the following questions and answer truthfully:

**Why am I dieting?** This one sounds obvious, but you might be surprised by your answer.

*Poor self-image? (I don't feel beautiful)*

*Trying to please someone?*

*Trying to fit into a pair of jeans or a favorite dress?*

*My high school reunion is coming*

*None of the above*

*Write your reason, here:*

_______________________________________

_______________________________________

_______________________________________

## Why am I overweight?

*Eating too many calories at each meal?*

*No exercise?*

*Poor food choices?*

*Larger body frame?*

*None of the above*

*Write your reason, here:*

_______________________________________

_______________________________________

_______________________________________

## Am I making lifestyle changes or temporary ones?

*Lifestyle changes          temporary (my dress...)*

*Explain:* _______________________________

___________________________________

___________________________________

___________________________________

## Is my solution practical (does it make sense)?

Yes        No

*Explain:* _______________________________

___________________________________

___________________________________

## Is my solution manageable (is it possible for me to accomplish)?

Yes        No

*Explain:* _______________________________

___________________________________

___________________________________

**Is my solution healthy and beneficial to me?**

Yes        No

*Explain:* ______________________________________

______________________________________

______________________________________

Our microwave society has lost sight of the nutrients of life that truly nourish and balance our bodies. Do you remember slowing down to enjoy a glowing sunset, enjoying a meal with loved ones or stopping to enjoy God's creation without feeling guilty about time? Constant dieting will not make for a healthy life. Eating consciously and simple lifestyle changes will create positive results and release you from the diet dictator's addictive, hungry maw.

Body balance can be achieved by evicting the

diet mentality and listening to what you truly need. Imagine taking all of the outward energy you expend on diets and fads and turning it inward, so that you can listen to your heart and that still, small voice. Enter less stress and a better way of life. There is no such thing as a quick fix. With careful thought and loving reflection, you can feed yourself in a nourishing way.

Working with your body, rather than against it, will bring you increased energy, stabilized weight and sustainable health. Develop eating patterns that are healthy and sustaining, and make them part of your daily existence.

The following questions relate to your health practices and general lifestyle. See how well you do on your responses:

1. How are your bowel movements?

a. How many movements do you have, daily?

b. Are they hard and hard to pass?

c. Are they really dark in color, and have a strong odor?

d. Do they look like pellets or a long, smooth shape?

2. How much water do you drink, daily?

a. Are you drinking at least one-half of your weight, in ounces?

b. Is the water room-temperature or always cold or filled with ice?

c. Are you drinking a glass of room-temperature or warm water upon awakening?

d. Are you drinking slowly, throughout the day or just gulping water when you remember?

3. What do your meals look like?

    a. Do you have fiber and protein at each meal?

    b. Are you avoiding liquids while eating?

    c. Do you have a cup of hot tea after a meal, especially one that has lots of grease and sauce?

    d. Are you eating lots of sweets and snacks?

4. What are your sleep habits?

    a. Do you have your last meal at least 3 hours before bed?

    b. Do you try to go to bed by 10:00 p.m., every night (or most nights)?

    c. Are you having at least eight (8) hours of sleep, nightly?

    d. Do you feel rested when you awaken in the morning?

Could you be sabotaging your weight?

*Doctor said it; I believe it*
*I don't question or object*
*I just take all medication*
*Even when I start to retch*

## Lie Number 4

### MY DOCTOR IS AN EXPERT AND, THEREFORE, KNOWS MY BODY BETTER THAN I DO

I don't want to question my doctor; he might be offended. I really should not question my doctor. I'll just do what he says. How many of us subconsciously nurture this lie? It is not a lie that most doctors are experts; rather, it is the latter half of the statement that needs reconfiguring. Your doctor is hardly the 'be-all and end-all' of all things symptom-related. Some of us have the tendency to listen to our doctors wholly, trusting implicitly and unquestioningly. He says it and we nod; he decides it and we agree; he writes the prescription and we open and swallow. We fear questioning him because we do not want to offend or insult; we prefer to offend or insult ourselves. Whose symptom is it, anyway?

No one knows your body like you do. You know what your symptoms are, the sensations, the joys and the pain. If you don't know yourself, then pay attention. Grab a mirror and examine your body; **all of it.** Examine moles, marks and lumps. Keep a journal and record your observations. You will also be able to note things that may have changed in shape, size or color, over time. Find words to describe the way that you are feeling. Don't gloss over how you feel; be vivid and accurate in your descriptions. In addition, use scales of one to ten to determine pain levels. If you develop the habit, then you will be able to accurately describe your symptoms to your doctor.

Remember though, that when you describe your symptoms to your doctor, you still need to listen objectively. Obtain a second opinion or a third, if need be; after all, *this is your life*. The cost of a co-pay or a fee for a second opinion pales in comparison to after-effects of hastily swallowed medication or the incorrect surgical procedure.

[*A little thing happened…*]

In 2012, my dermatologist prescribed antibiotics (Doryx) for a horrible facial infection that I had developed after visiting a spa. Knowing how sensitive my body is to drugs and how long it had been since I had even taken Tylenol, I told her that I am not in the habit of taking medication. She told me to try it and see if it would help my skin. Truth be told, she did not need to persuade me too much; my face looked like I had leprosy or a nightmarish case of chicken pox. I forgot myself in the face of my desperation. People had started to recoil when they saw me.

On the second or third day of the medication (I had been given a 12-week supply), I noticed slight stomach cramping. I ignored it for a few days, during which time the pain increased. I started taking it on alternate days. It did not help because by the time the pain abated sufficiently on my off-day, it would return, in full force, on medication day.

When the pain travelled to my left side, I called the doctor. She told me that I could stop taking the medication and she would give me a different one. I refused it. My pharmacist, with whom I have a good relationship (long story), told me to get over the pain and take the medication because it was for my good. Really! I knew, then, that I needed to do that which I should have done all along – take the healing of my skin in hand.

I increased my greens and started making more green smoothies. I made poultices with neem powder or moringa powder and bentonite clay. I drank moringa mixed in water or smoothies; I juiced more, used more turmeric and other beneficial herbs, and kept myself properly hydrated. Soon, my skin began to come out of hiding. Soon, my stomach stopped hurting. Soon, I felt less embarrassed. Soon, people stopped recoiling when they saw me.

What additional lesson did I learn? Well, a few weeks after my experience, I was searching for something and came across a little pouch with the Doryx. I had taken the drug before. It was several years ago and although I believe that I had written down my reactions, I did not add Doryx to my computer file with all the others, so I had no basis for a stronger refusal to the dermatologist. Of course, I now keep all of this information in one place. I could have hurt myself even more than I had.

Listen to your body. It is your only house and you can't sell it or exchange it for a newer model. Speak up when you do visit the doctor. Do not be afraid to ask questions and take notes. Ask doctors to spell words with which you are unfamiliar.

Research them. There is too much information on the Internet for you to claim ignorance. Just type the name of the medication and you can narrow the search by typing "What is…?" or "Side effects of…" in front of the title. Ask about the necessity of prescriptions, the side effects and the difference between generic and original brands. Ultimately, you are the one who needs to live in the house, so the renovations must be appealing to you.

*I care for my family,*
*my own health can wait*
*I have obligations, there is no debate*
*Not feeling so well, now*
*I'll give it some time*
*It's selfless to put their needs above mine*

## Lie Number 5

### MY FEELINGS CAN WAIT; TAKING CARE OF OTHERS IS MORE IMPORTANT

Before we even talk about physical symptoms and signs, let's talk about stress. Most women internalize our worries, our fears, frustrations, and our hopes because expressing them causes us to be labeled as 'drama queens' or being 'emotional' or 'melodramatic.' What do we then do? We hide.

Everybody comes to you with problems or to vent but no one seems to have time to hear yours. We do like to hear that we are 'great listeners' though. All that you have done is add to your burden. It does not mean that you ought not to listen, but you then need to let it go, rather than add their issues to your back. Mothers tend to do this a lot, especially with adult children. Tell, me- how is this helping you?

Let me be presumptuous and answer for you. It is not helping you. Did you know that, over time, stress can make you physically ill? Diseases like cancer, diabetes, migraines, stomach problems and issues with the thyroid and heart are exacerbated by stress? For a more detailed explanation of that, read my book, *When Stress Comes to Stay*[8]. In it, I show you exactly what you are doing to your body by having Stress as your houseguest.

Many women may feel pain or a strange sensation in their bodies, and they dismiss it to focus on all that they have to do and be. They delay investigating, sometimes, until it is too late to do anything about it. I wonder why it is that we do this. Some of it, I know, is the result of being too busy. Some is cultural bias; women are not as important, a lie we have come to believe, too. Some reasons, though, are a little more self-serving.

It seems that we live in a society where having something about which to complain actually provides fodder for social situations. Some of us seem more apt to dwell on the things that are

---

[8] *When Stress Comes to Stay*, Lesa Lawson, ND. Available on Amazon.com

wrong. Have you ever attended a party or gathering of any kind where the conversation shifts to someone who is ill or who has pain or a lump or some other affliction? Given time, during the conversation, other people will chime in with woes of their own to outdo the one who has spoken.

All in all, we sometimes do not check these signs or symptoms until they become difficult to ignore. Why wait until the hour is late? How does that help you? Go and check. Find a clinic if you do not want to go to the hospital. Talk to a qualified professional. Am I encouraging hypochondriac-type behavior? Not at all; I am simply appealing to the part of us that understands responsibility, a responsibility that ought to extend to ourselves.

Thinking of your own health does not make you selfish. What's the point of discovering conditions when it's too late to do anything about them? Even if you place others' needs above your own, will you be able to serve if you are ill? We teach responsibility in more ways than we realize. Our children watch us; indeed, their strongest lessons are learned when they are simply observing us. If we don't take care of ourselves, we are teaching them to do the same. We are telling our girls, especially, that their health is not important, either.

I figure that we would like to enjoy our lives for as long as God allows. Let's live it in the best way that we can, with the best health that we can maintain.

*Thin is in; that's what they say*
*Grab the scale and start to weigh*
*One-ten! Oh, my word, I'm fat*
*What will my friends say about that?*

## Lie Number 6

**WE HAVE TO BE THIS THIN TO FEEL BEAUTIFUL.**

I have been trying to figure out when this hype started; the hype of the thin woman. Natalie Wolchover, in her article called "The Real Skinny:

Expert Traces America's Thin Obsession,"[9] dates the beginning of the fascination between 1890 and 1920. At that time, plump women began to be associated with slothfulness. Since then, we have gravitated towards certain models and actresses as our role models for thinness.

We perform self-flagellation, hating ourselves because we are not all size ones or zeros. This awful feeling then transfers itself into our behavior, which we then pass on to those around us. Soon, everybody around us begins to reflect our mood, which then makes us feel even worse about ourselves and our treatment of them. By this time, our guilt swells to anger, and so the cycle

---

[9] *The Real Skinny: Expert Traces America's Thin Obsession*, Natalie Wolchover, Life's Little Mysteries Staff Writer. Date: 26 January 2012 Time: 09:58 AM ET

continues. Maybe we should add 'masochist' to the list at the beginning of this book!

There is a difference between being at an unhealthy weight that stems from improper foods, little exercise, insufficient sleep and lack of hydration, versus having a larger size because that is your body's frame. Every woman does not have to look like the model in the title. If you look closely enough, you will see that she's emaciated, looks malnourished – okay, she's a skeleton. The last time I checked, people avoided skeletons.

We're not all supposed to look the same. Examine yourself. Look at your height, your frame, your diet, your sense of happiness, and your overall outlook. If there is something that you are not doing, and you know that you ought to, then do it. Do not complain that your thighs are bulky if you are not walking or doing some other form of exercise.

You may need to change your dietary habits, so begin. Some of you are bombarded by so many options and programs, that you do not know where to start. If you are uncertain about where you are, or if you are ready to make the change from dieting to living, contact me. There are some suggestions in the next chapter that may be of help.

## ALL TRUTHS

## EIGHT EASY STEPS TO JUMPSTART YOUR HEALTH BREAKTHROUGH

Having explained that many of us women are selfless to the point of self-neglect, I know that all of us will not always make a miraculous, instantaneous mental turnaround. For some, I know it will not be that easy. Some things were easy for me to change but some were challenging and took a lot longer than I would have liked. Still, we are works in progress.

We listen to the voice of our heavenly Father because He is always telling us how to care for ourselves. Sometimes, He will send you help; Enter Dr. Lesa Lawson to the rescue.

You may not know how to take time for yourself, or how to listen to your body's signals. You may acknowledge that the information herein applies to you, but you are at a loss as to what to do next. Solution: Contact me for a 30–minute discovery session to help you devise a strategy for self-care (See my information on the last page of this book).

Here are eight steps that you can incorporate into your life. They will help to bring clarity. Remember – you are a beautiful child of God, a child whom He desires to bless and see at peace, and well.

**Try to have...**

**One** mental health day per week (or at least one hour) Relax...

**Two** servings of fruit, daily (try something new, each week)

**Three** days of exercise (20 minutes. Walk up and down your stairs, or through the mall. Walk with a friend)

**Four** servings of vegetables, daily (at least).

**Five** minutes of reflection, daily. Start a "thankful journal."

**Six** scriptures or words of encouragement to tape to your mirror, fridge door, wall... Repeat them to yourself, aloud.

**Seven** morning meals (Not seven meals a day but rather, have breakfast everyday)

**Eight** glasses of water, daily (at least 8; regardless of what you hear).

# On a Personal Note

Dear Friend,

Do you know that God wants you to be well and at peace? He loves you so very much. His Word, the Bible, reveals His love and yearning over you.

*"The LORD has appeared of old to me, saying: 'Yes, I have loved you with an everlasting love; Therefore, with loving-kindness I have drawn you.'" Jeremiah 31:3 (NKJV)*

He wants you to be well in your mind, body, and spirit. He wants you to care for your body with proper exercise, diet, and rest; He wants you to take care of your mind by alleviating stress, and addressing emotionally oppressive issues.

*"Guard your heart above all else, for it determines the course of your life." Proverbs 4:23 (NLT)*

God also wants you to take care of your spirit. He invites you to share a personal relationship with Him through His Son, the Lord Jesus. If you have not met Him, know that this can only be done by accepting Jesus Christ as your Lord and Savior.

Pray this prayer to Him, in truth:

Dear God,

I believe that You love me and sent Your Son, Jesus Christ, to die for my sins. Thank you for forgiving me and I ask You to take control of my life. I give myself to You. I look to You to help me and lead my life; in Jesus' Name.

**Congratulations and welcome to the family!**

If you don't have a Bible, try to obtain one or read from your cell phone. The Bible is God's love letter to you. Talk to Jesus, your new best friend, often, about any and everything. Ask Him to lead you to a church, where you can learn more about Him.

# ABOUT THE AUTHOR

Lesa Lawson, ND is a Naturopathic Doctor and certified Colon Hydrotherapist. Her practice is firstly, integrative (blending age-old healing traditions with scientific advances and current research). Secondly, it is holistic (treating with a number of mental and social factors which impact human health negatively).

Dr. Lawson specializes in alternative therapies that help clients regain their digestive health. Her area of focus is the gut / stomach as it is the seat of most illnesses arising from factors such as poor diet, dehydration, medications interacting negatively with one another, stress, or unhealthy working or living environments.

Her personal and professional health journey led to a profound appreciation for healing from the inside out. Dr. Lawson's learning in alternative medicine began quite unwittingly as a child, at the feet of her parents in her homeland of Jamaica, West Indies. That interest grew when as an adult she battled personal health challenges and learnt of illnesses that family and friends faced. She continues to do research in Jamaica and in the United States.

Not satisfied simply with apprising herself of information and because her practice is one in which she, along with her clients, are partners in their health, she educates readily, and has conducted seminars in Jamaica and the United States.

Dr. Lawson is a member of the American Association of Drugless Practitioners (AADP) and the International Association for Colon Hydrotherapy (I-ACT).

She carries her own line of products such as Moringa Blend, CholestCheck and Gentle Clean. Services include colon hydrotherapy, botanical recommendations, magnetic analysis, and 90 and 120-day weight, nutrition and wellness programs

She is the founder of LawsOnHealth Wellness, a haven of healing located in Northern Virginia. Dr. Lawson's first work is the thought-provoking, *Six Lies Women Believe about Their Health*, followed by *When Stress Comes to Stay*.

Lesa Lawson, ND, CHC

Naturopathic Doctor
Colon Hydrotherapist

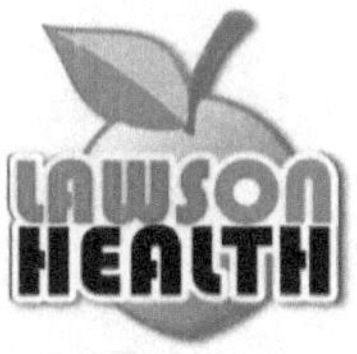


LawsOnHealth Wellness Center

(571) 252-3428

E-mail: lawsonhealth@gmail.com

Website: lawsonhealthwellness.com

# Products

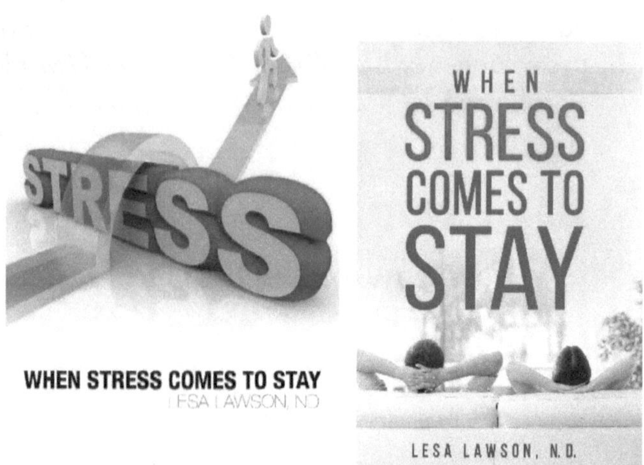


***When Stress Comes to Stay***, Dr. Lesa Lawson
Order: Amazon.com

**Nature's Sunshine:**
https://www.naturessunshine.com/us/
*receive 33% discount with $40 purchase and account*
Sponsor number: 794343

**dōTERRA**®: *Essential Oils*:
http://mydoterra.com/lesalawson
ID#: 1175848

**Kangen Water Machines** (*Alkaline Water*):
www.enagic.com
Distributor ID: #615755